Optimal Brain Health

Care for Your Brain's Health to Ensure Optimal Brain Function and Performance!

Ron Kness

Published by:

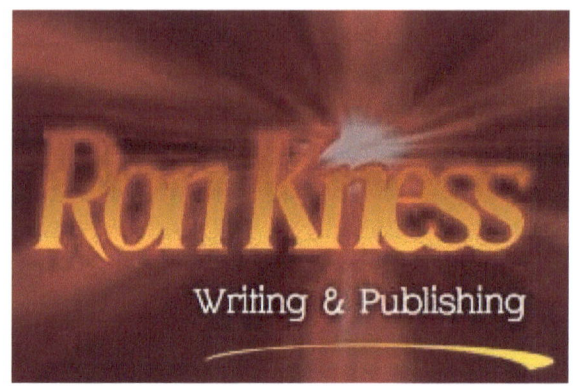

https://ronknesswriting.com

Ron Kness

San Tan Valley, AZ

United States of America

ISBN: 9781095217719

Optimal Brain Health
Contents

Introduction

We would all like to have 'perfect health'. That is, every part of us working exactly as should, with no illness or dis-ease.

Although for most people there is little value in trying to quantify it, some parts, systems and organs are more critical to our health and even our very survival than others.

Taking this to the limit, there can be little doubt that the most critical component of all is the brain.

We tend, naturally, to often think of our brain in terms of our ability to think and reason – the 'higher functions' that seem to set us apart from others in the animal kingdom.

However, our brains perform myriad functions autonomously, automatically and subconsciously that affect the health and wellbeing of our entire body.

Yet, when people think of their health, they all too often think of the physical health of the rest of the body. Or they may think of their emotional or mental health, but not really take into consideration the need for caring for the physical health of the brain, as an organ.

This book provides enlightenment regarding the health of this most vital organ. It discusses how some of our modern lifestyle aspects are detrimental to our brain wellness, and how to moderate their effects.

A major part of the book is devoted to practical and proven ways to help your brain stay healthier. In doing so, you will be 'starting at the top' in improving your overall health and wellness.

The Importance of Silence to Brain Health

Your brain needs silence. Perhaps not all the time, but your brain cannot be healthy and productive without it.

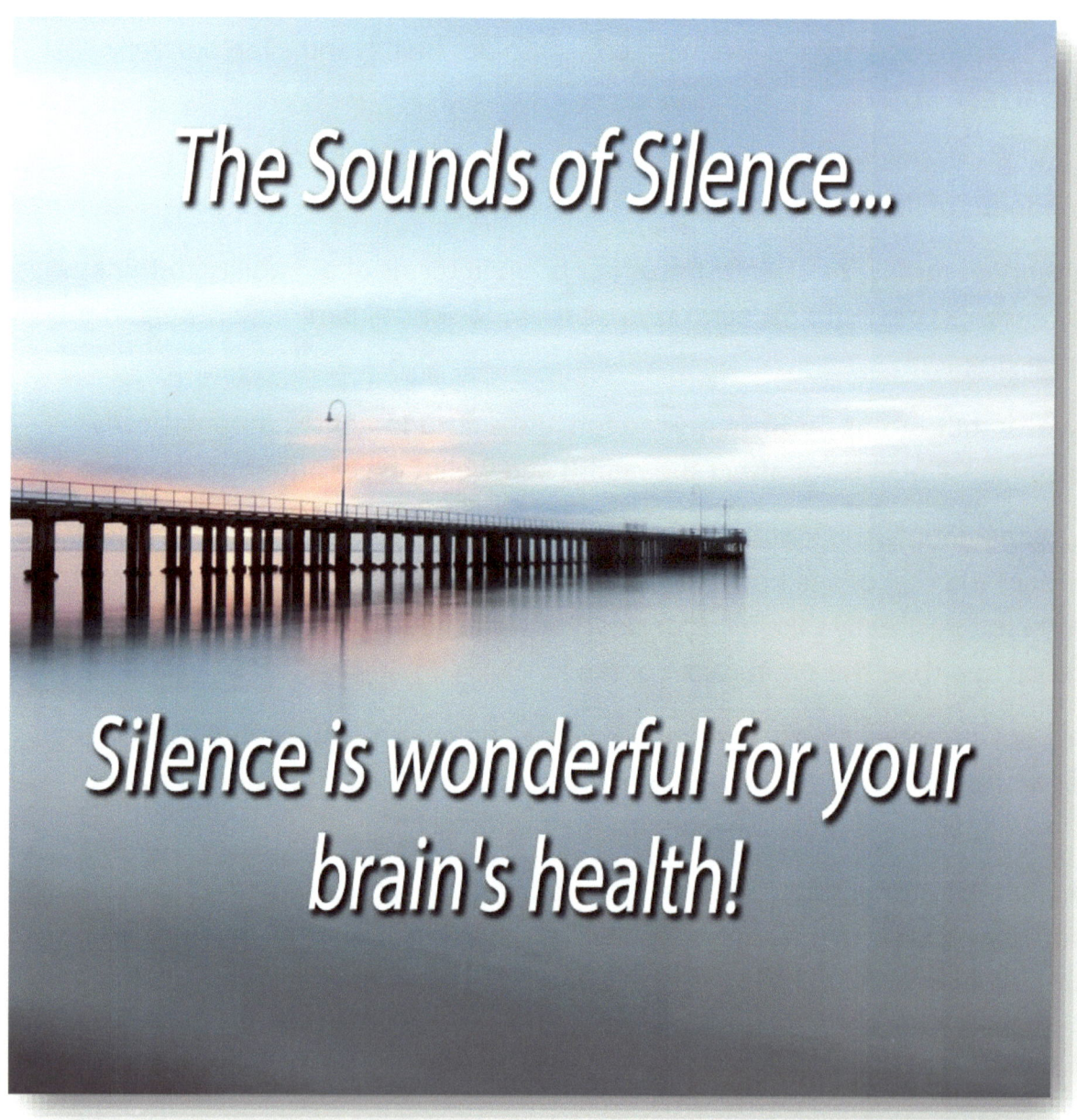

The Sounds of Silence...

Silence is wonderful for your brain's health!

There are many benefits to 'the sounds of silence', such as triggering the development of new brain cells and enabling the brain to actually 'think' (as opposed to just carrying out its untold number of automatic processes).

Silence Triggers the Development of New Brain Cells

Studies show that silence helps trigger the development of new brain cells which develop into functioning neurons. The hippocampus, which is responsible for learning and for processing emotions and memory, shows newly developed cells after exposure to silence.

Silence Enables the Brain to Think

Some people believe that silence relaxes the brain too much, whereby it becomes unproductive. This is not entirely true. If you are in a totally silent environment the brain is still busy processing thoughts and busy sorting and evaluating information.

You would have experienced this, by silently pondering and reflecting on past events. When your brain is not distracted by noise, it can smoothly process information.

Noise Stresses the Brain and the Body

Noise can have a negative impact on the brain, resulting in the body releasing the stress hormone cortisol. Experts believe that the amygdala, which is situated within the brain's temporal lobes, is constantly activated through the chronic production of the stress hormones.

The amygdala is the part of the brain responsible for processing memories and emotions. Therefore, an individual living in a noisy environment is more likely to release chronically high levels of cortisol.

Even if the level of noise does not produce hearing damage, it may certainly be loud enough to cause 'dis-stress' on the body, both physically and mentally, as a result of this constantly-engaged brain activity.

Silence Releases Stress from the Body

If noise is a problem, silence is a solution. Silence helps release stress from the body.

The findings of a study which was published in the *Heart* journal showed that two minutes of silence provided more relaxation benefits than a person listening to two minutes of music.

Noise Harms Cognitive Functioning

Noise is also harmful to a person's productivity and performance. It decreases motivation while increasing the tendency to make mistakes. Noise can have an adverse impact on the brain's cognitive functioning and affects the brain's ability to process memory, solve problems, and focus.

Noise Increases Risk of Illness

Experts have discovered a link between high levels of blood pressure and chronic exposure to noise from airports or highways. It has also been linked to higher rates of heart disease, tinnitus and sleep loss. These studies were performed in an effort to show how 'noise pollution' has a negative effect on health.

As we said earlier, noise leads your body to produce the hormone cortisol. This significantly strains your body's entire system, resulting in elevated blood pressure levels and heart rate, while chronically constricting blood vessels. This is a precursor for developing heart disease.

It also can increase the risk of developing anxiety and depression and unwanted behaviors such as anger and aggression.

To better understand the impacts of noise on our heart health, a study showed that being exposed to persistent noise greater than 65 decibels, did indeed affect the cardiovascular system.

- 65 decibels is similar to that of the background noise in a restaurant.
- 85 decibels is approximately the level of noise a blender makes.

How the Brain Reacts to Music

Numerous studies have been conducted to show how something invisible to see, such as noise, can create such a profound effect on a person's physical wellbeing.

When noise is heard, its sound waves reach the ear as it vibrates through the cochlea. The cochlea converts these sound wave vibrations into electrical signals so that the brain can process them. Even when you are asleep your body reacts to these electrical signals in the brain, even in a deep sleep cycle.

Neurophysiologists say that the sound waves from noise are first activated in the amygdala. This is where numerous clusters of neurons activate to process memory and emotion.

As far as reacting to music, study participants were asked to listen to 6 different musical tracks. They found that the music manifested changes in each person's blood pressure and carbon dioxide, and also in the brain circulation. For each sound track, there was a corresponding physiological change that occurred.

The most interesting finding was observed between the musical tracks. The blank pauses in between tracks suddenly became the object of their study. They found that the silence gave study participants a release from carefully paying attention to the music they were listening to and provided a deeper sense of relaxation.

What to Do to Turn Down the Noise

If you live where it's noisy, you can improve your surroundings with several tweaks. For example, make your home more soundproof by filling any holes or gaps to the outside. You can also change your windows, and also hollow doors with solid ones, to help soundproof your home.

If internal noise in your home is higher than you'd like it to be, perhaps turn off any devices when you're not actively paying attention to it, such as the TV and music players.

Sleep Cleans the Brain

Have you ever wondered why you need to sleep (and not just because you know you have to in order to survive), but really ever wondered the real 'why'?

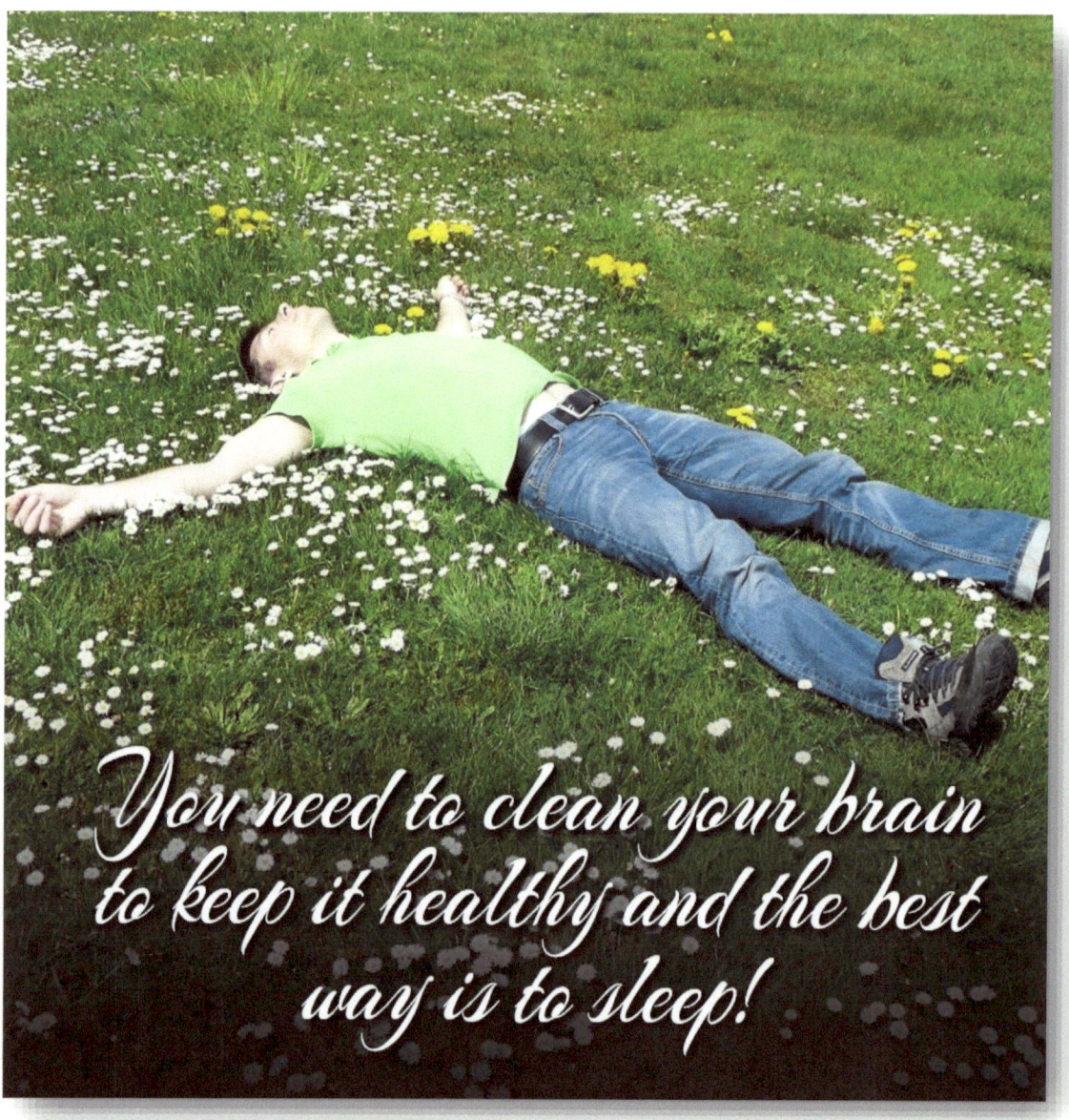

You need to clean your brain to keep it healthy and the best way is to sleep!

If asked why we do, most of us wouldn't be able to give the correct answer, in regard to the importance of sleep and how it impacts brain health.

Your Brain Cleans Itself While You Sleep

During sleep, your brain cleans out all the toxins that have accumulated while you're awake. The cellular structure of the brain changes during sleep. One study published showed that the brain cells shrink during sleep, creating gaps between the tissues, allowing the neurological waste to be passed out and flushed away.

This waste removal system of the brain is what experts refer to as the glymphatic system. This glymphatic system has been found to be ten times more active when a person is sleeping.

The brain flushes the waste through its cerebrospinal fluid. The same fluid is responsible for bringing in nutrients to the brain.

Getting Enough Sleep Lowers Your Risk of Alzheimer's

This cleaning process does more than get rid of toxins. Another important reason to get plenty of sleep is to enable the brain to flush out beta-amyloid proteins.

If your brain is healthy these proteins are flushed out easily, however, if it isn't healthy, these beta-amyloids can accumulate as sticky plaque and cause problems. The plaque has been found in larger amounts in patients diagnosed with Alzheimer's.

If you don't get enough sleep, your brain cannot do its cleaning process which can result in the accumulation of neurotoxins such as beta-amyloid proteins.

More Beta-Amyloid Problems

Another study was aimed at determining how sleep can help prevent the onset of memory impairment. One of the findings suggested that the beta-amyloids played a role in preventing a person from getting enough sleep.

This in turn triggered the onset of chronic sleep deprivation.

Neuroscientist Matthew Walker, one of the experts involved in the study, found that having an increase of beta amyloids in the brain led to the increased likelihood of not being able to achieve deep sleep. It also impacted on memory.

Unfortunately, the less sleep you get, the less capable your brain is in cleaning out the beta-amyloids, and the vicious cycle begins where your brain health can begin to deteriorate.

Bedtime Habits that Harm Your Brain

Neuroscience experts suggest that people pay better attention to their sleep hygiene. Factors such as diet and exercise are certainly important for enabling the body to get enough sleep. However, there are other, more specific, bad habits that can hinder quality sleep.

For example, sleeping with a smartphone close to your head adversely affects certain patterns of the brain. Smartphones emit signals that have the capability of adversely restructuring brain cells and preventing the process of cleaning out neurotoxins.

The electrical radiation that is emitted from smartphones and other mobile devices is picked up by the brain. Although scientists are still trying to determine just how much damage wi-fi gadgets are causing to the brain, it's safe to say that removing them from close proximity is a good habit to get into.

In doing so, you are giving your brain the chance to clean itself, and also getting quality sleep that is essential to physical health too.

Sleep, Even If You Don't Feel Sleepy

Quite often you'll hear people say how they don't need a lot of sleep, yet they are still capable of doing what is required of them. Unfortunately, even if a person does not feel sleepy, they need to go to sleep! The brain needs at least 6 to 8 hours of sleep each night for it to be able to get rid of the neurotoxins.

Plus, whether a person believes it or not, a well-rested brain is far more capable of performing optimally than one that is sleep deprived.

If getting enough sleep at night is a challenge for you, take the time for a 20-minute nap during the day. Taking a nap is like recharging your smartphone battery. It boosts your brain's memory and learning capacity.

For people who can nap for an hour or even 1.5 hours, they are able to help their brain build new connections, which translates to improved creativity.

Although many people would like to believe that the brain has unlimited powers, research suggests otherwise. Experts have found that the brain has limitations.

For example, it cannot perform its daily tasks while doing its housekeeping. It either needs to work or clean. Therefore, if you want to keep a healthy, clean brain, let it do its job when it needs to and go and get some sleep!

Do You Know the Signs of Mental Fatigue?

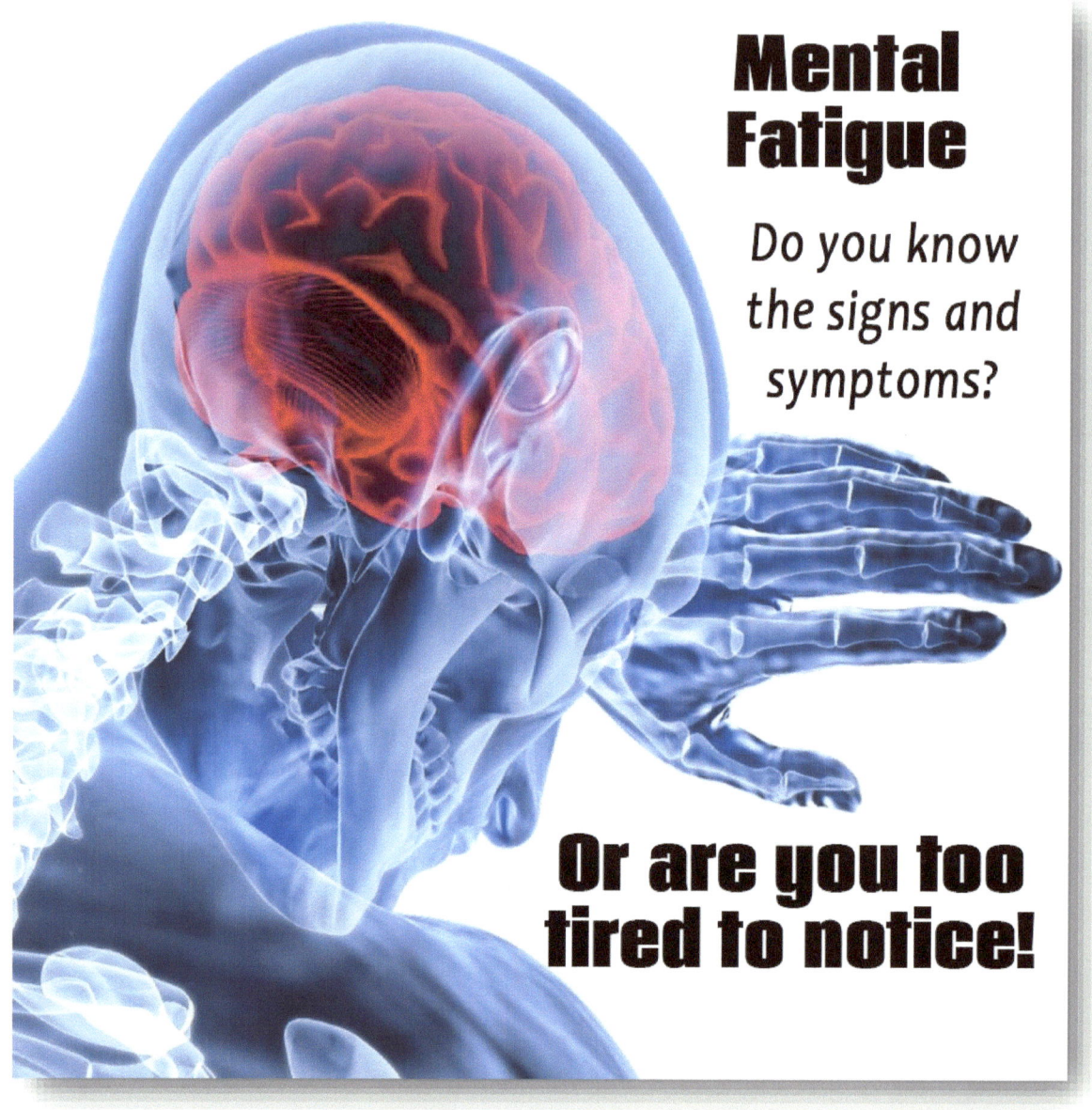

Mental fatigue occurs when the brain is overstimulated, or through a lack of sleep and/or suffering from chronic mental stress. If a person is mentally stressed, they may find it hard to get to sleep and/or stay asleep, or alternatively, stressed individuals may require more sleep than usual.

Healthy sleep is crucial for physical and mental health, so recognizing the signs of mental fatigue is important.

Memory Retention Problems

If you are lacking sleep your brain may become much less capable of retaining information. It may be retaining some, but not all. It just isn't as affective as if you were getting quality sleep. Therefore, if you are having problems recalling or retaining vital information, you may be showing signs of mental fatigue.

Brain Feels Foggy

Think of your computer for a moment. If you have too much going on, everything slows down or freezes. It needs to shut down and have a restart. It's as if your computer has mental fatigue. The same applies to you.

If there's too much going on your brain must deal with the overload and may begin to feel foggy. If you are showing signs of brain fog, it's time to shut down, take a sleep and recognize this sign of mental fatigue.

Easily or Often Confused

People suffering from mental fatigue become easily confused especially when bombarded with an overload of information. They tend to struggle with coping with all the sensory inputs being sent to the brain.

An example of being confused through mental fatigue, is the need to have someone repeat themselves, even though you heard perfectly. You just didn't take it in. Your mind was elsewhere and not focusing on the task at hand.

No Longer Feeling Motivated

If you are mentally fatigued the last thing you will feel is motivated. If you are battling to get out of bed to want to start your day then mental fatigue is hitting you hard. No motivation is a big warning sign!

Highly Emotional

If you are feeling irritable, anxious, sad, and just not in the mood to do anything, you are quite possibly showing signs of mental fatigue. Out of control emotions are a sure sign something is up, whether it be stress hormones kicking in or mental fatigue. Either way, it's time to calm down and relax.

Change in Eating Behaviors

Mental fatigue may drive a person to indulge in and crave sugary or salty foods, while others may suffer a loss of appetite. Eating too much (especially of these poorer food types) or too little is not good for you.

These negative eating behaviors are signs that your brain is not coping with all the stress it is dealing with, so it's time to make changes.

Physical Aches and Pains

Your mind and body are connected, therefore if your mental health is having problems, your physical health will begin to show problems too. If you are beginning to experience muscle pains, headaches, constipation or high blood pressure, then you may be suffering from mental fatigue.

Mental fatigue may manifest physically in some of the following forms: rapid heart rate, fainting, shortness of breath, stomach pain, or teeth grinding. These signs are letting you know that your body is not working harmoniously with your brain.

Remember it's your brain that is the central processor of the entire working systems of your body. Therefore, a healthy brain is a vital part of a healthy body. Make sure your brain health is performing optimally so that your entire body is performing the best it can too.

How Stress Affects Brain Health

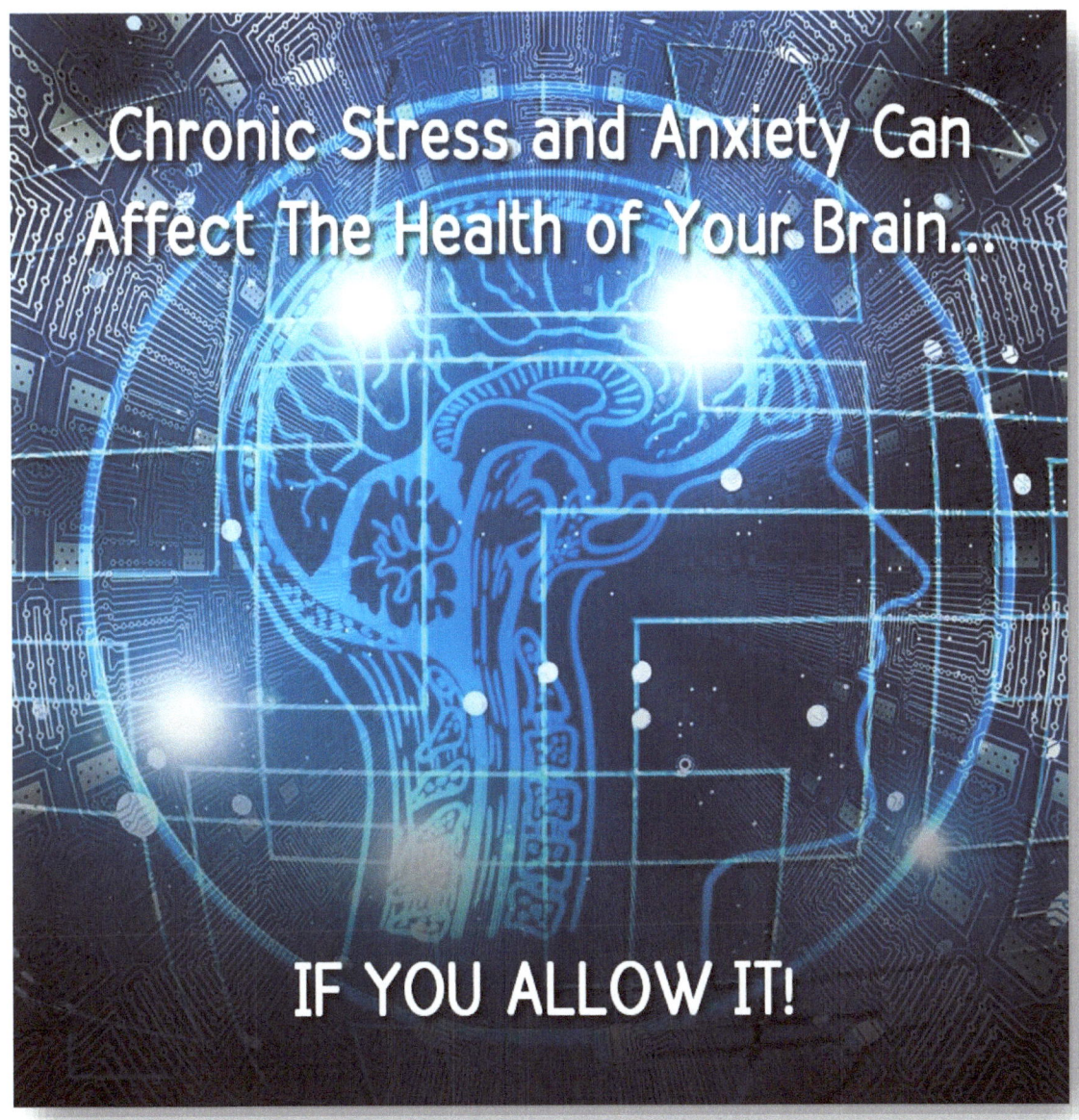

It's probably fair to say that most people feel some degree of stress and anxiety during their day. It certainly doesn't feel good at all. Needless to say, we need to reduce the stressors in our life as much as possible or we run the risk of harming our physical and mental health in many ways.

We all feel an anxiety response to any threatening situation and the body is ready to fight or flee. This response causes the body to produce norepinephrine and cortisol.

These stress hormones power up the body's senses so that perception and speed are improved in the immediate short-term. The heart rate quickens, and the body is ready to act! However, if stress like this is put on your body continually, after a while it takes its toll.

The Differences Between Stress and Anxiety

Let's look at the differences, as you may be putting stress and anxiety into the same basket, and it can be difficult to distinguish between the two. At first glance, anxiety does look a lot like stress.

Experts explain that anxiety may occur as a result of undue stress. Stress certainly can make a person feel the same symptoms: sad, depressed, anxious or fearful, which are the same as anxiety.

However, the cause of the anxiety may not be apparent. Someone with anxiety may not know why they feel that way, whereas stress can be caused by many factors in the person's environment. Therefore, stress can be caused by external influences, while anxiety is an internal response.

Chronic Stress Changes Your Brain

Prolonged exposure to stress triggers the creation of hard-wired pathways located between the amygdala and hippocampus. These newly created pathways can predispose a person to constantly suffer from stress.

The amygdala is the part of the brain which plays a crucial role in helping the brain process sensory signals. The amygdala is responsible for quickly alerting the brain of an imminent threat. This triggers the brain, producing an anxious or fearful response.

The hippocampus is responsible for encoding memories. Evidence from studies show that people who have experienced abuse or traumatic events have a smaller hippocampus. This is because prolonged exposure to acute stress shrinks the hippocampus.

Chronic stress also leads to a reduction in the number of stem cells. Unfortunately, these stem cells are crucial for a person's memory and learning.

This explains why chronic stress makes it hard to absorb new information, while also causing a decline in memory. No wonder a stressed-out person finds it hard to remember things and is said to be forgetful. They may regularly misplace their keys or forget appointments.

Chronic Stress Causes Brain Cells to Die

If chronically stressed, the hormone cortisol is produced. This production triggers the creation of a glutamate surplus which also causes free radicals. These free radicals have been found to attack the cells of the brain.

This attack is like oxygen attacking a metal that results in the metal rusting. These free radicals create holes in the cell walls, and ultimately causing cell death.

Stress Inhibits the Production of New Brain Cells

We all lose and produce brain cells daily. A type of protein called BDNF, or Brain Derived Neurotropic Factor, plays an important role in helping the brain produce new cells and making sure the brain cells are healthy.

Some experts refer to BDNF as the brain's fertilizer. It can offset the adverse effects of stress on the brain.

However, chronic stress, which makes the body chronically produce cortisol hormones, can inhibit BDNF production. This results in the low production of new cells. Studies have shown that low levels of BDNF are linked to dementia, Alzheimer's, depression and OCD.

Severe Stress Increases the Risk of Toxins in the Brain

Your brain has a semi-permeable filter commonly referred to as the "blood-brain barrier", which is a group of cells.

These cells perform a special task that allows nutrients to enter the brain, while making sure that harmful substances don't. Severe stress can weaken this barrier and pathogens, harmful chemicals, toxins and heavy metals may enter the brain.

Can Your Brain Health Recover?

The brain possesses the natural ability to recover from damage caused by chronic stress. Once the stressors are removed, the neural stem cells can begin once again, to normally produce new neurons.

If you feel you are suffering from too much stress and anxiety and are worried about what it's doing to your brain health, don't give up!

There are ways you can relax and regain a sense of calm.

Effects of Cell Phone and Wireless Waves on the Brain

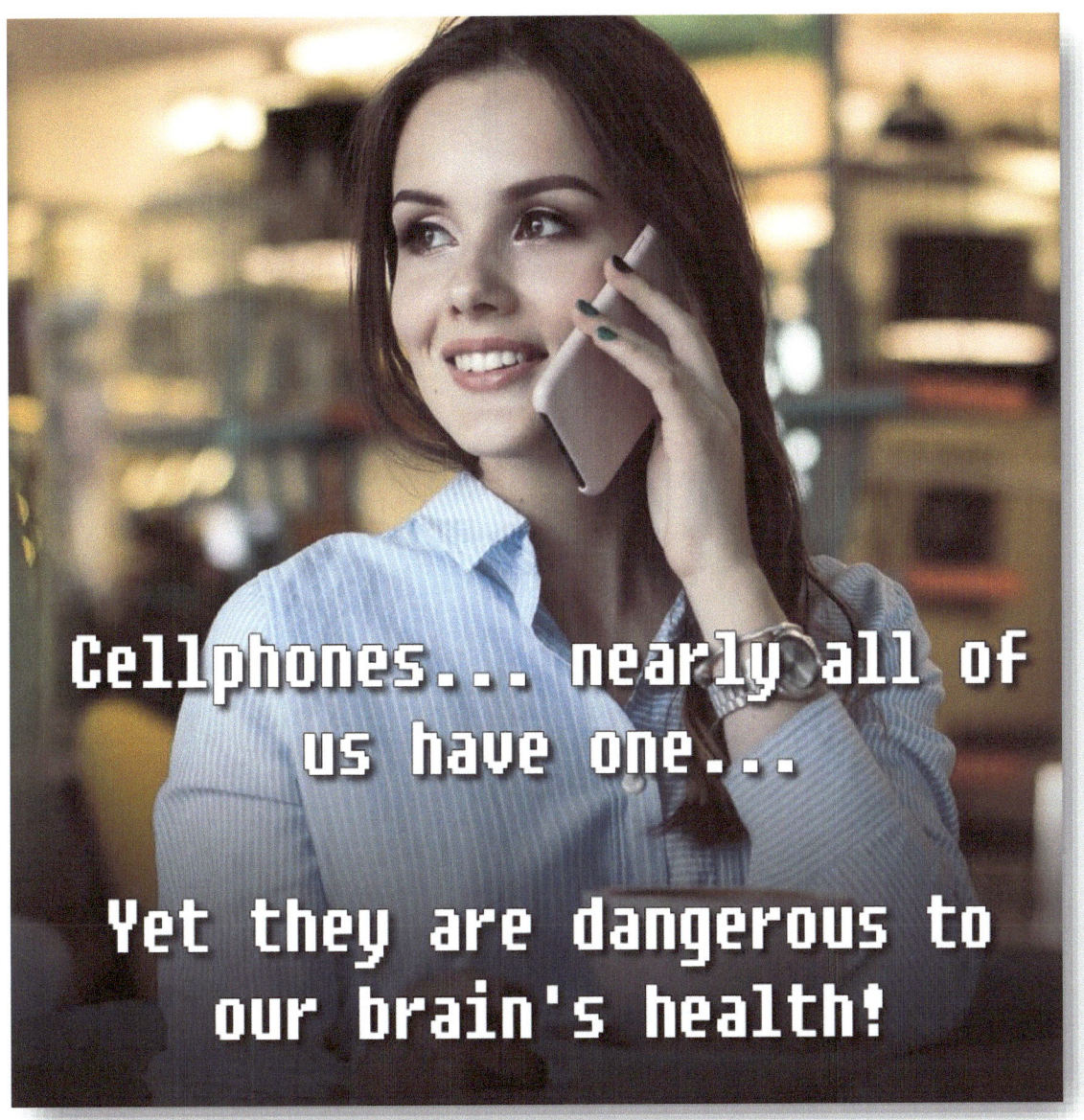

Cellphone use has been linked to the increased risk of brain cancer, because of its ability to change brain activity. However, cellphones harm brain health in many ways! Cancer is just one problem.

This article presents several findings from studies, which show how cellphone use and the exposure to wi-fi signals affect the brain.

The cells inside the brain communicate through electrical impulses. These impulses can be detected via a non-invasive EEG or Electroencephalogram device.

A study of participants who underwent exposure for fifteen minutes to a 3G mobile phone, showed cortical reactivity in the brain significantly increased soon after exposure to radiation.

This study is not the only one that suggests that acute exposure to cellphone radiation can indeed have negative effects on the brain.

Another study revealed that the brain's alpha band (i.e. EEG pattern) changes when exposed to cellphone radiation.

It Alters Glucose Metabolism in the Brain

Yet another study, published in the *Journal of the American Medical Association*, suggests that using a cell phone for 50 minutes results in the alteration of glucose metabolism in the brain.

This change was seen in the area of the brain closest to where the cell phone antenna was placed. This effect of cellphone usage was seen using a PET or Positron Emission Tomography scan.

To date, there is no known safety level of exposure to cellphone or wireless radiation.

Although these studies show how the brain reacts to cellphone radiation, more research is still needed to be able to determine the exact health consequences.

Researchers stress that even though at this time they may not be able to accurately quantify the potential damage, the point that has been made clear is that the human brain is sensitive to mobile phone radiation.

Effects of Mobile Phone Usage

For the past ten years, the number of people developing cancer has increased. Data collected from studies has led to claims that this increased rate of cancer is correlated with the prevalent use of wireless devices.

The evidence showed that people who hold their cellphones close to their face were at a higher risk.

Cellphone and other wireless gadgets are known to release intermittent pulses of radiation which have been found to cause disruption to human DNA.

In addition, this erratic microwave radiation emitted from mobile phones has been found to weaken the protective barriers of the brain, which can trigger the release of highly destructive free radicals to enter the brain.

Another study showed that the cerebral blood flow in the brain changed when exposed to cellphone radiation.

Children Are More at Risk

In one of the issues of *San Francisco Medicine* magazine, Dr. Devra Davis from the Environmental Health Trust stated that children are more prone to the effects of cellphone radiation.

For example, a child who is only five years of age does not yet have a fully developed brain. Experts have said that the bone marrow in the child's head was found to absorb radiation ten times more, compared to that of an adult's brain.

Tips to Reduce Health Risks from Cellphone Usage

You can take precautionary measures to reduce your risks and protect your health.

- Use a headset when you need to use your phone. A headset keeps your ears, head and face away from the radiation, which is strongly emitted while the phone is active.

- Use non-metal cases. The non-metal cases don't transfer the radiation as much as the metal ones do.

- Turn off your wireless router when you're about to sleep. This reduces the likelihood of your brain and body absorbing radiation while you're sleeping.

- Eat plenty of healthy green vegetables to boost your body's ability to naturally repair radiation damage.

How Sugar Affects the Brain

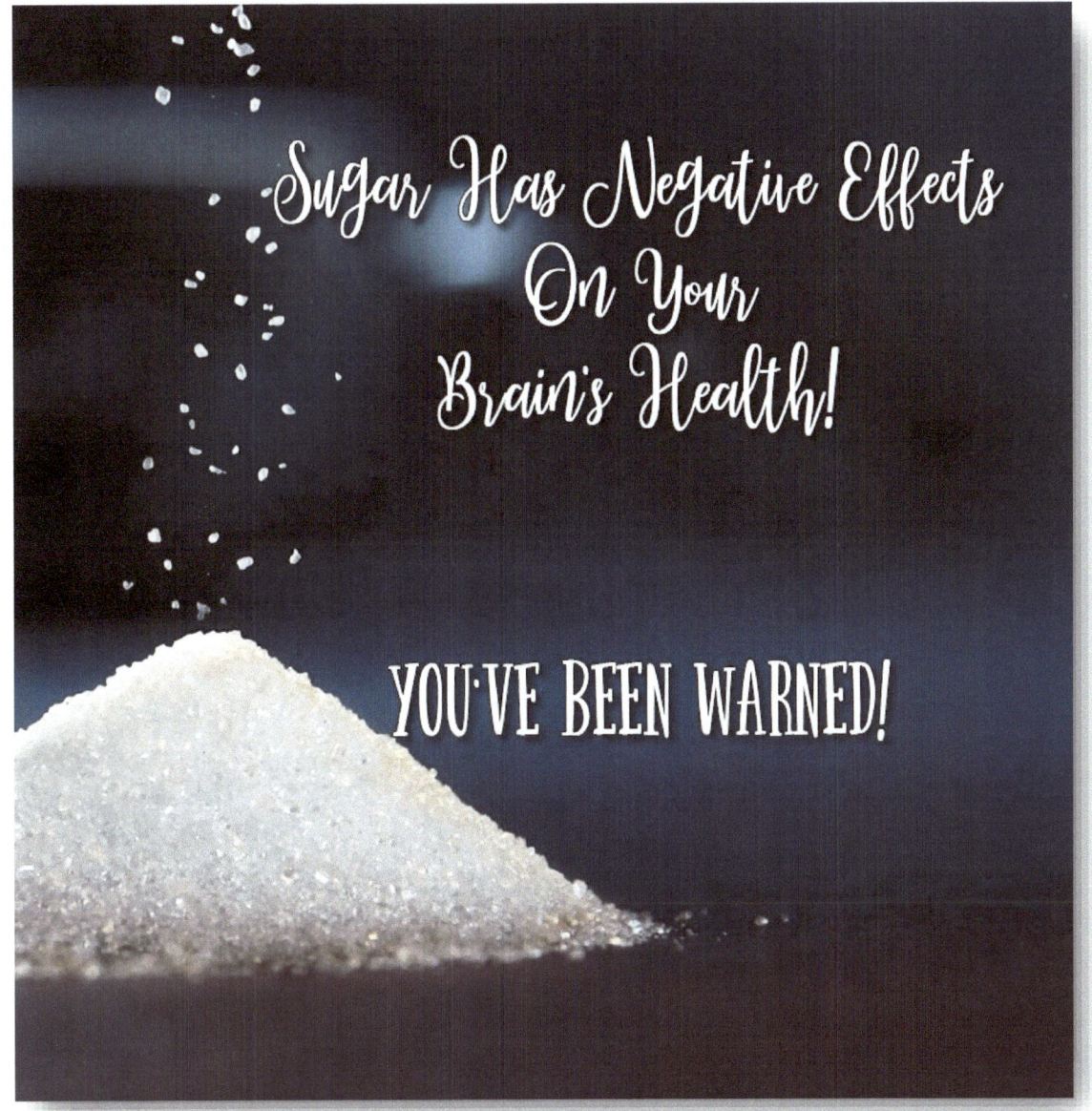

If we eat or drink a sugar loaded product, our taste buds and brain instantly acknowledge the sweetness. For most of us a sugary treat tastes good!

Unfortunately, if we allow ourselves to eat sugary-laden foods all the time, our health will suffer, including our brain health.

The moment your taste buds recognize the sweetness, the brain is signaled.

The reward pathways in the brain light up, triggering the release of dopamine – your happy hormones. This is why you feel good when eating something sweet.

The problem is, if you keep eating sugary foods, your brain's reward system will be chronically activated. This puts you at risk of craving these types of foods every day, or as often as possible. You crave a sugar hit!

This is when you start to lose control and your body develops an increased intolerance towards the amount of sugar that you consume. If left unabated, you can develop a sugar addiction and will undoubtedly give in to all your cravings.

As neuroscientist Nicole Avena said, an over stimulated reward system of the brain will trigger the occurrence of several adverse reactions in your brain and body.

Sugar and Your Brain's Neurotransmitters

Eating sugary foods leads you to experience a sugar crash. Soon after eating sugar, whereby you may feel a rush of energy, the 'crash' occurs. This crash occurs as a result of your blood sugar levels plummeting. This is due to a panic release of insulin, as your body tries to protect itself from the influx of sugar.

This sugar crash manifests in the form of brain fog, irritability, fatigue and a change in mood. Once your body's glucose levels dip, you are bound to feel moody, depressed and anxious. You may also feel suddenly very tired and want to lay down.

Part of the reason why this negative reaction occurs is because the sugar adversely affects your brain's neurotransmitters. Not only does the sugar release dopamine, the excessive sugar consumption leads another hormone, serotonin, to be excessively produced as well. Once this hormone becomes depleted, your happy mood is depleted too.

Your sugary treats can have you twirling around in a vicious cycle, whereby you simply crave sugar again to boost your moods once more.

Sugar Increases Risk of Cognitive Decline

Studies show that excessive sugar consumption slows down the brain and affects memory and learning.

Regular, excessive sugar consumption leads to the development of insulin resistance. This then leads to problems regulating the body's blood sugar levels, and therefore increases the risk of developing diabetes.

Insulin plays a crucial role in strengthening the synaptic connections in between the cells of the brain. This is critical for better communication between the neurotransmitters and memory.

Once insulin production dwindles, cognitive processes may also suffer. Evidence strongly indicates that the brain is one of the main victims of high sugar consumption.

Sugar Can become An Addiction

When you consume sugar, the prefrontal cortex becomes activated and your feel-good hormones, such as dopamine, are released. This sends a signal to your brain that it should remember this great feeling. As with any addiction, this is how it begins. It's a 'want more of' feeling.

Sugar also activates the brain's *nucleus accumbens* which is the pleasure center. If it is turned off, this is when the person may develop depression, alternatively, if it is stimulated, by consuming sugar for example, then 'the want more of' (addiction of the substance) may begin.

As this cycle occurs, the signal being sent to the pleasure center becomes weaker. This makes you consume even more sugar in order to feel that wonderful experience again.

As you can see, the sugar consumption is no longer filling the void it once did, and the more it is consumed, the more health issues arise.

The reason it becomes an unhealthy addiction is because the sugary foods leads the brain to create a path that becomes easy to activate. This newly developed path or circuit serves as a shortcut to pleasurable feelings, each time sugar is consumed.

Unfortunately, this circuit will eventually become the brain's default path, and this translates to addiction.

Chronic consumption of sugar foods can also cause your brain to not recognize signals that you should stop eating. The sugar dulls the signals the brain's need to keep you and your body healthy.

This is in part because excessive sugar consumption leads to the reduction of oxytocin, which plays a role in preventing binge eating.

There lies the vicious cycle to a sugar addiction and the health of your brain.

The more you eat, the more you crave, and the more you eat the more damage to your brain's health.

Brain Exercises – Keep Your Brain Healthy

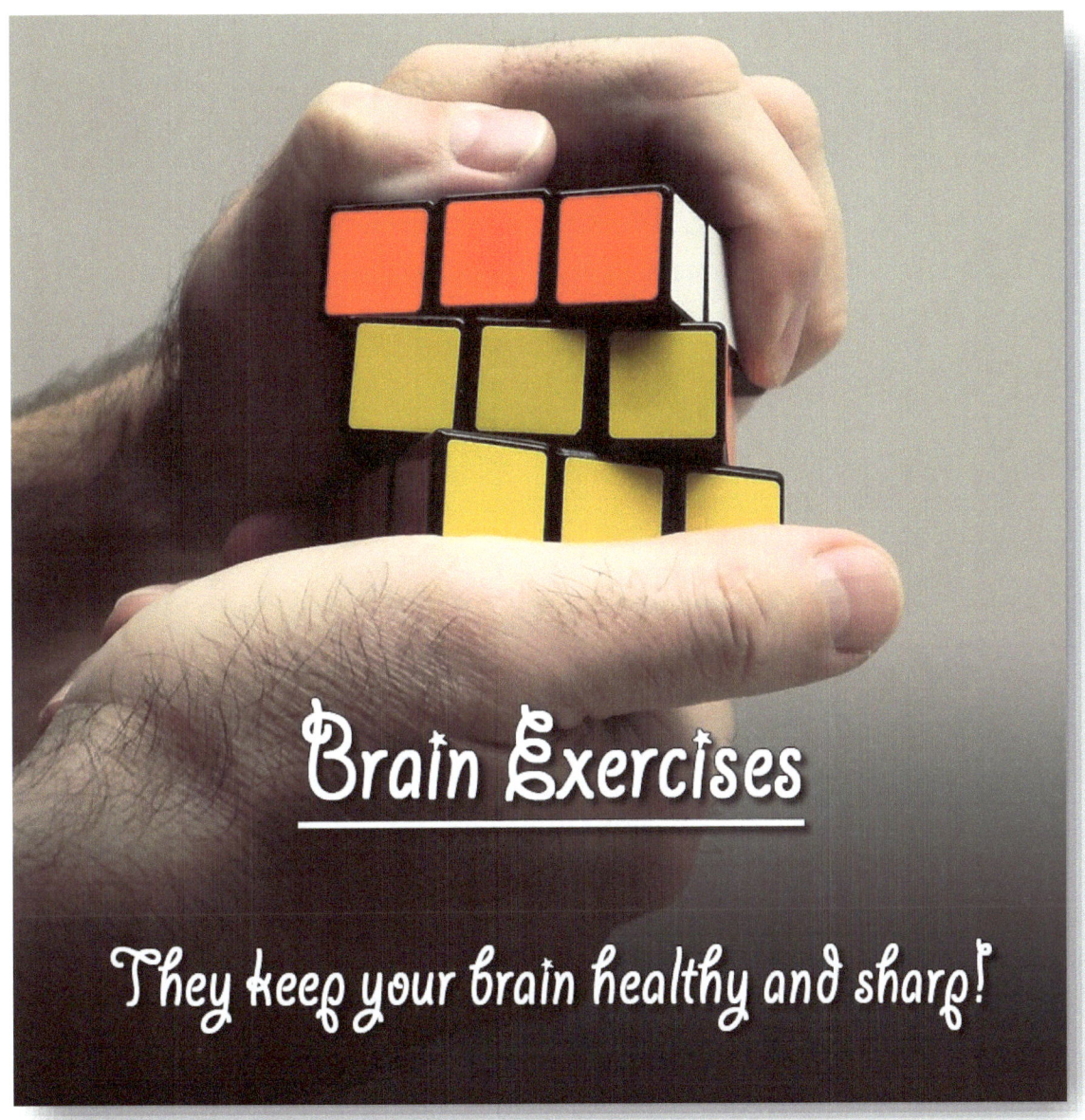

Although physical exercises such as running and jogging are good for your brain health, there are other exercises you can do while sitting to make your brain healthy, sharp and smarter.

Here are a few brain health exercises you can do.

Observation Exercise

You can do this alone or with a partner. While sitting in a public place memorize the details of the people you see. You can start with memorizing three details, then progress to memorizing more. If you're with a partner, make it a game and take turns to see who remembers the most details.

This exercise is what brain experts refer to as 'passive memory training' because it doesn't warrant any special memory techniques. It simply allows the brain to indulge in a fun activity, rather than make it perform at its peak and store the memories in its memory bank.

If you want to become a better observer, this exercise will certainly help you develop memory skills. You can also try this exercise on cars or buildings or any objects for that matter.

Play '10 Things'

This brain exercise is where you take an object and try to think of '10 things' that may be similar to your object. Take an egg flip for example. What other things are similar to your egg flip? Is your brain working in over-drive wondering what else it could be? Or did you think of 10 things easily?

If you can't think of any, how about a guitar, or a shovel, or even a fly swatter. Now it's your turn to come up with a few more! As you can see a game like this forces your brain to really think hard and makes it stronger.

Indulge in Art If You Don't Already

Drawing or being creative artistically is a relaxing brain exercise, and therefore has the added bonus of providing relief from stress. A brain that suffers less from the impacts of stress is not just smarter but healthier too.

It also makes you use the creative side of your brain. You may not do this every day, but investing some time on art projects can greatly improve your brain's ability to process nonverbal and emotional cues.

It's Time to Start Reading Aloud

Reading aloud allows your body to use other brain circuits. This is the reason why many editors and writing experts recommend that reading aloud should be done during the editing process.

When each word is spoken out loud, the brain 'can hear' the dialogue or conversation. This enables the brain to easily pick up grammatical errors etc. It also helps improve the memory as you are far more likely to remember what you have 'said and read', than just read.

Other Brain Games

This article wouldn't be complete without mentioning the Rubik's cube. This is one brain exercise that can either frustrate you or have your brain trying as hard as it can to solve the puzzle! If you can, congratulate your brain! Well done!

As for other ideas, there are plenty of things you can do to exercise your brain and boost its power. The key is to allow your brain to try out new, novel and complex things.

If you do, new neurological pathways will develop inside your brain. The more you engage in brain exercises the less likely your brain will decline in cognitive function.

Plus, a smarter brain boosts your self-confidence, speeds up your reaction time and enables you to think faster when you must.

Relax Your Brain with Meditation

Meditation allows your mind to focus and relax. Meditation causes you to focus on your breathing, thoughts, and the sounds around you, or you can focus on whatever you want.

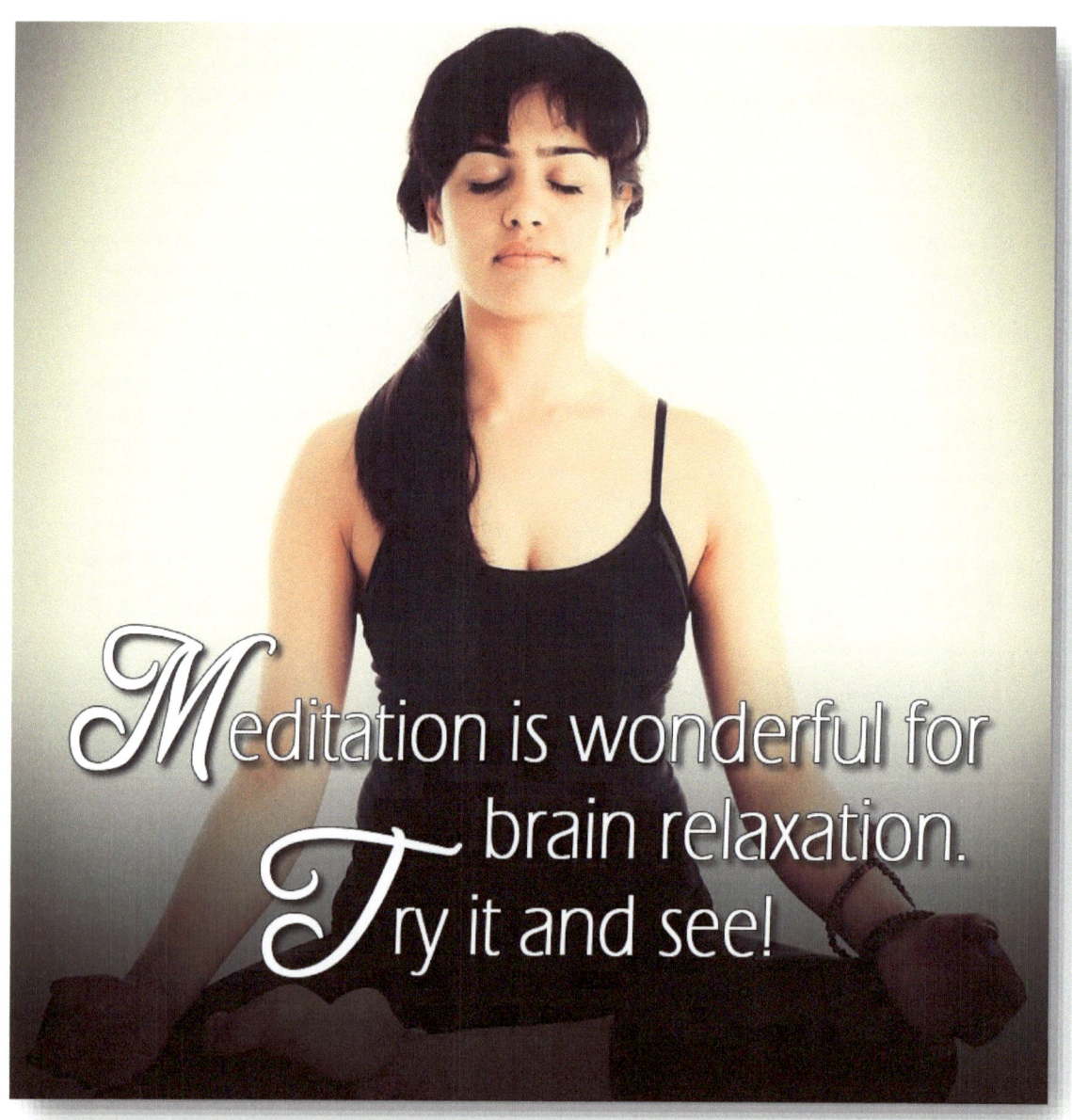

Meditation is wonderful for brain relaxation. Try it and see!

By directing your conscious mind to focus on specific targets, it distracts, or prevents it from 'churning', 'ruminating' or 'planning' types of brain activities.

Our modern lifestyles cause our brains and minds to be constantly bombarded and overloaded with sensory input.

Considering the degree of data overload most humans experience, it is not at all surprising that chronic stress affects as many people as it does. Simply stated, we did not evolve to deal with level of constant brain engagement.

Meditation provides an antithesis to this frenetic, unnatural activity. Meditation allows your brain to relax, which is why it is so beneficial for your brain's health.

Meditation Helps Ease the Distressed Mind

Meditation has been used to help patients suffering with emotional stress and also anxiety. Many people have had success from their mental anguish after practicing mindfulness meditation for one hour a day over an eight-week period.

Meditation used in conjunction with other relaxation techniques such as yoga and other gentle exercise, have proved to be even more helpful. A study was performed to determine the effects of mindfulness meditation. Each study participant had a brain scan done before and after the mindfulness session.

The scans showed increased activity after the session, compared to before the session. This increased activity was found in the area of the brain responsible for processing information.

The results also showed that their amygdala, the part of the brain responsible for processing anxiety and stress, became less active. This translated to reduced feelings of anxiety and stress.

Meditation Reduces the Size of Amygdala

Another study suggests that meditation helps the brain's amygdala become smaller. Stress, anxiety and other forms of emotional trauma have been found to enlarge the amygdala, and the larger it is the more reactive it becomes.

This particular study used participants who were suffering from extremely high levels of stress. All of them were asked to undergo mindfulness meditation practice for eight weeks.

After their mindfulness meditation training, the participants' brains were found to be more resilient and less reactive. Plus, they had reduced feelings of stress and anxiety.

Meditation Increases GABA Production in the Brain

Another study revealed that engaging in meditation and yoga helps the brain to produce more gamma-aminobutyric acid or GABA. GABA is a neurotransmitter in the brain and many people suffering from anxiety issues, show low levels of this neurotransmitter.

There are prescription medications and natural supplements designed to help increase the production of GABA.

Regardless of whether you attend classes to learn how to meditate, or you practice mindfulness meditation at home, the results are the same. Your brain will relax and your health will reap the benefits.

Therefore, take some time out of your busy day and give your brain the chance to relax and find some peace. It will make you feel a whole lot better!

Health Foods for Your Brain

It's no secret that the foods you eat contribute to your total health and wellbeing, and that also includes your brain health.

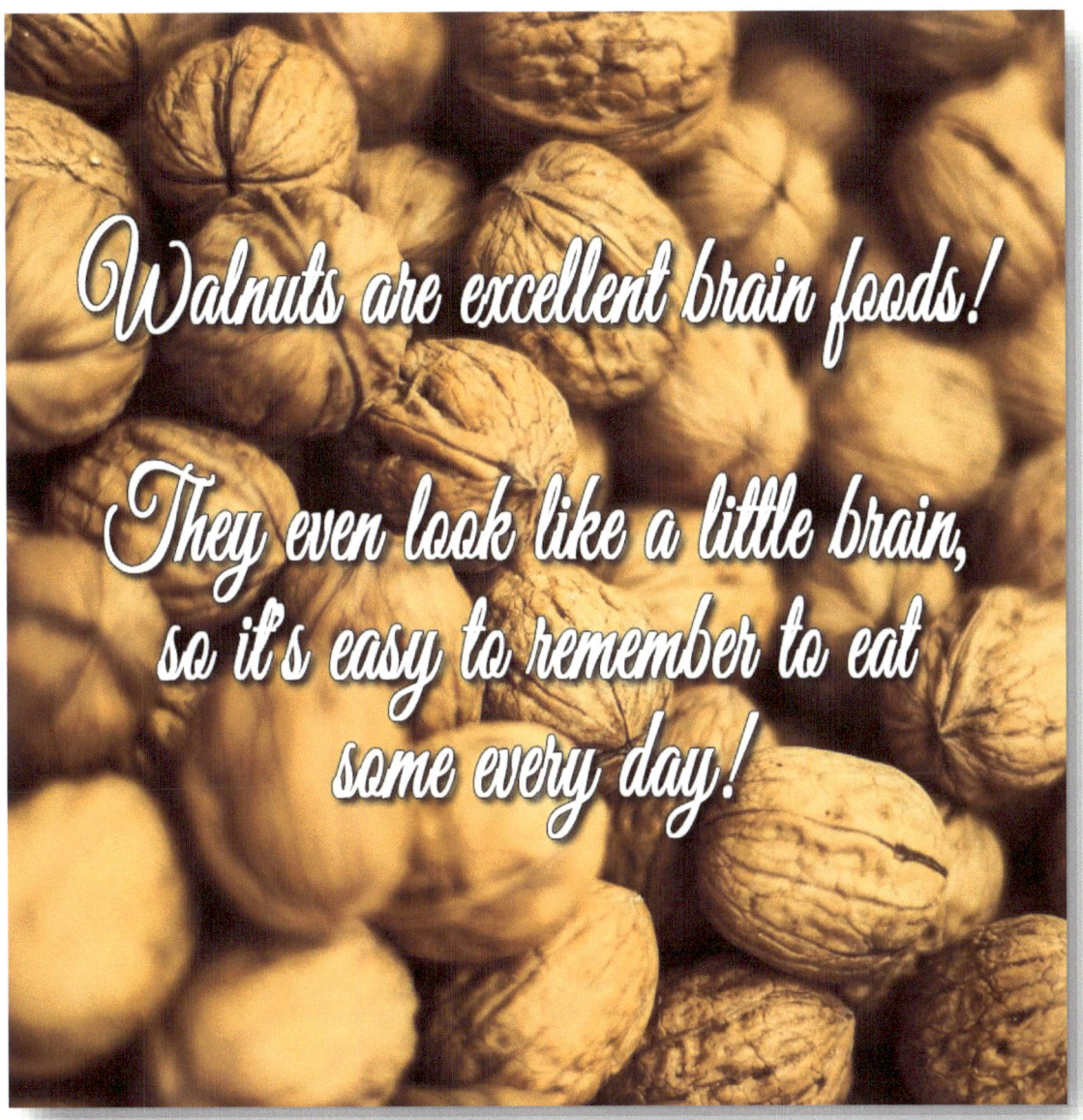

If you'd like to take better care of your brain health, you can start right now with these brain-nourishing foods.

Walnuts

The first one on our list is easy to remember because it looks like a little brain! This brain 'look-alike' food is the walnut. Walnuts contain many nutrients including vitamin E and have been found to be help improve memory and brain function. So, if you want to take care of your 'nut' eat approximately 7 walnuts daily!

Wild Salmon

This deep-water fish has earned a healthy reputation for being rich in omega-3 fatty acids. Omega-3s help keep the brain cell membranes healthy while also aiding in the formation of new cells. Omega 3s are also important for reducing inflammation and assist nerve transmission. If you can add 3 x 4-ounce servings of wild salmon a week to your diet, your brain will thank you.

Avocados

The brain needs healthy fats to function at its best, so eating avocados is a great place to start. Avocados contain monounsaturated fats that promote a healthy flow of blood to the brain. They also contain potassium which is important for blood pressure regulation and Vitamin K is another essential nutrient found in avocados.

Beets

Beets contain a high nitrate content. These natural nitrates are converted by the body into nitric oxide which promotes oxygenation all throughout the circulatory system. Studies have shown that the consumption of beet juice leads to an increase in oxygenation to the brain. More oxygen to the brain boosts cognitive function and reaction time. It also improves the neuroplasticity (or the neural pathways) of the brain.

Eggs

Eggs are full of protein which is important for the production of essential neurotransmitters such as norepinephrine and dopamine. These neurotransmitters largely contribute to feelings of alertness and improved energy levels. Eggs are definitely a superfood.

These little powerhouses also contain B vitamins, such as folic acid, B12 and B6. These B vitamins play a crucial role in reducing the amount of homocysteine in the blood. High levels of homocysteine have been linked to cognitive impairment, Alzheimer's disease and stroke.

Broccoli

One cup of broccoli gives you more than 100% of your daily requirement of vitamin K. This fat-soluble nutrient plays a significant role in the formation of sphingolipids which are fats found in the brain cells. Vitamin K helps promote better memory and it helps to fight against inflammation which protects the brain from degeneration.

Broccoli also delivers sulforaphane which has anti-inflammatory and antioxidant capabilities, which help promote the development of brain tissues. Sulforaphane is also found to be beneficial for repairing damaged brain tissues.

Dark Chocolate

If you don't like broccoli, perhaps you like eating dark chocolate. Dark chocolate is full of flavonoids which are important for healthy brain function. They assist with boosting memory and learning processes. Flavonoids also help slow down the decline in mental skills as we age.

Another important aspect of brain health is our moods. The consumption of dark chocolate has been linked to improved moods. It tastes good and makes us feel good, as it promotes the production of 'feel-good' endorphins. It also has a naturally-occurring compound called anandamide which is referred to by experts as the 'bliss molecule'.

Of course, with anything that tastes good, eating dark chocolate in moderation is key! You don't want to become a 'chocaholic'!

Vitamins Needed for Good Brain Health

Vitamins are important for the body's nourishment and normal growth and are required by the body in small but essential quantities from dietary sources.

There is no other organ in the body that requires as high a concentration of vitamins and minerals as the brain. Why? It's because of all the work it does! It has many, many tasks to perform 24/7. It never takes a break.

Therefore, if you want to keep your brain functioning at an optimal level, make sure you get enough of the following vitamins. There's nothing more powerful than a brain running on all cylinders!

Vitamin D

Vitamin D is famous for its ability to promote better bone health. However, few people realize its crucial role in brain health. Vitamin D helps with managing moods, blood circulation and memory function.

A vitamin D deficiency is linked to many problems in regard to mood, immunity, attention and sociability.

Vitamin D helps with basic cognitive functions being performed. One study involving mature adults showed that having higher levels of vitamin D led to improved cognitive function.

So, if you want to give your brain a boost, make sure you get plenty of vitamin D, by getting out in the sunshine and/or through your dietary sources. Foods containing vitamin D include eggs, sardines, salmon and tuna.

Vitamin C

The human brain is composed of around 86 billion neurons that help transmit information via neurotransmitters. Vitamin C plays a crucial role in the production of these neurotransmitters which have a significant impact on the way you sleep, focus and remember things.

Besides assisting in the production of neurotransmitters, vitamin C helps protect the brain from free radical damage.

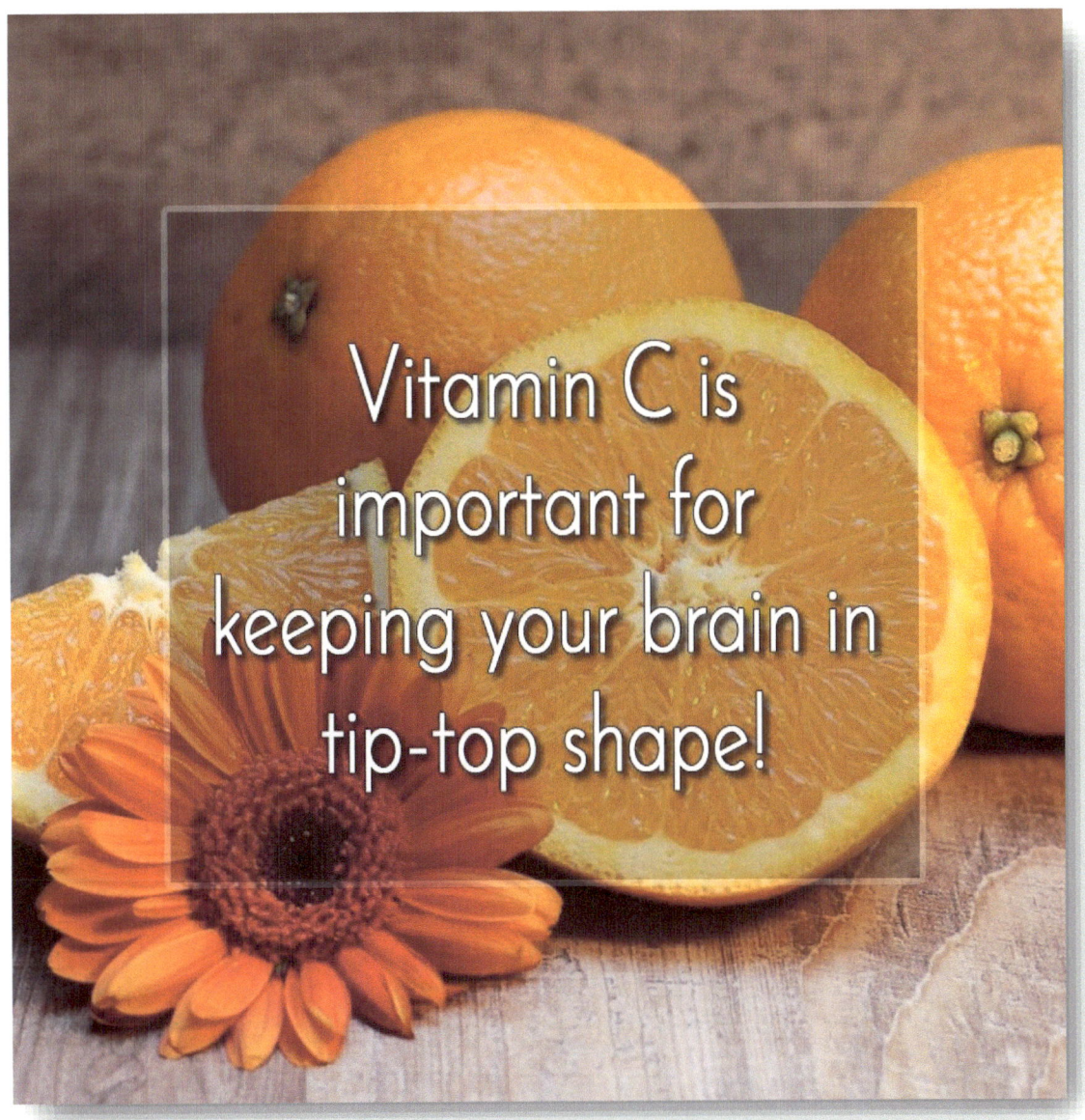

Vitamin C functions as a potent detoxifier. It can enter the blood-brain barrier and remove toxic metals from the brain. Experts suspect that these metals in the brain are part of what is causing problems such as Alzheimer's disease.

Vitamin C also improves blood flow to the brain, keeping it well-nourished with increased levels of oxygen and nutrients. Guava, black currant, red pepper, kiwi and orange are few of the many best sources of vitamin C that you can eat daily.

Vitamin E

The brain needs a sufficient supply of vitamin E. This fat-soluble vitamin is an antioxidant that has protective effects on the brain. It is known to protect cell membranes from the adverse effects of oxidative stress.

Unfortunately, the brain is highly susceptible to free radical damage and the risk increases as a person ages. The effects of free radical damage have been found to be the main contributor of neurodegenerative diseases.

A deficiency of vitamin E may result in problems with balance and coordination. It can also lead to abnormal eye movements.

Vitamin E also helps in the prevention of Alzheimer's disease and has also been found helpful in slowing down the progression of the disease.

Sunflower seeds, wheat germ, hazelnuts and almonds are some of the best sources of this essential brain healthy vitamin.

Vitamin B1 or Thiamine

Vitamin B1 has a critical role in the maintenance of several brain functions. The brain needs energy. It is a huge energy-consuming organ of the body. The brain actually requires one-fifth of the body's overall energy supply for it to be able to function at full force. This is where vitamin B steps in.

Vitamin B serves as the cofactor - a non-protein chemical compound which is needed for enzyme activity - to millions of energetic reactions taking place in the brain.

For example, if you need to burn glucose for energy, you need thiamine to make it happen, and glucose is one of the most important energy sources for each brain cell.

Vision impairment, brain fog and dizziness are some of the symptoms of a vitamin B1 deficiency. Seaweed, macadamia nuts, sunflower seeds and lentils are good sources of thiamine.

Vitamin B9 or Folic Acid

One study shows that high levels of folic acid in the body helps slow down cognitive decline among the aging population. Folic acid is essential for DNA and neurotransmitter health.

It also aids in cellular detoxification as well as healthy functioning of the nervous system. It plays an important role in amino acid synthesis for proper nerve tissue development.

Although it is primarily recommended as being an important vitamin for pregnant women, folic acid is crucial in all ages and genders. A deficiency of this vitamin contributes to the onset of vascular dementia and Alzheimer's disease.

In a separate three-year study which had more than 800 participants aged 50 and above, it showed that those participants who took folic acid supplements had better scores in their memory tests. These results were comparable to people more than five years younger than the study participants.

Excellent sources of folic acid include dark green leafy vegetables, asparagus, broccoli, okra and avocado.

Make sure you add plenty of healthy foods mentioned above to provide your brain with the necessary vitamins it needs for healthy brain function.

Conclusion

We shouldn't need to be told of the importance of our brain health. But, it is not the sort of thing we sit and ponder over every day. We all have too many other things to do.

It is not possible to overstate the importance of having a healthy brain, yet most of us are neglectful in this area. Of course, some of our efforts to improve our health in other areas do thankfully contribute to the health of this precious organ.

On the flip side, our brain's health, or otherwise, has huge impacts on all areas of our health and wellbeing.

By following the recommendations in this book, you will be able to improve your brain health, which will be a very big part of achieving a healthier, happier you.

Referenced Books

The following books referenced in this book are all Printed Paperback Perfect Bound form:

Cortisol - https://www.amazon.com/gp/product/153978598X

Heart Disease - https://www.amazon.com/Heart-Health-Lifestyle-Putting-Factors/dp/1511940476

Sleep Hygiene- https://www.amazon.com/gp/product/1790401585

Sleeping Clean - https://www.amazon.com/Sleeping-Clean-Healthcare-Improve-Restful/dp/1729453872

About the Author

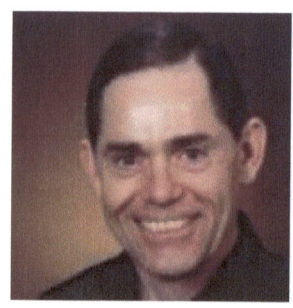

I have published numerous books on Amazon (both for Kindle and in paperback), along with other publishing platforms.

While most of my books are on health and fitness in general, I also write on baby boomer and older citizen health issues and have a recent interest in creating and printing journals/ planners and other printable products. A complete list of our published products on Amazon can be found at https://www.amazon.com/Ron-Kness/e/B0072M6PYO.

Besides my own writing, I also ghostwrite ebooks, books, reports, articles, blogs and do Kindle conversions for clients on a variety of topics. Contact me at Ron Kness Writing for a quote.

Today my wife and I are retired from our careers and live in San Tan Valley, AZ. I now write as a retirement business where you'll find me happily sitting in my office typing away on my laptop as I work on my next book or ghostwriting project . . . that is if we are not traveling on a cruise ship - our new-found mode of travel.